Interstitial Cystitis Cookbook & Meal Plan

Simple and Appetizing Recipes to Alleviate Discomfort, Fix Pelvic Floor and Bladder Issues, and Reclaim Your Quality of Life.

Title:
Interstitial Cystitis Cookbook & Meal Plan

Subtitle
Simple and Appetizing Recipes to Alleviate Discomfort, Fix Pelvic Floor and Bladder Issues, and Reclaim Your Quality of Life.

Printed in the United States of America.

ISBN: 9798876028129

TABLE OF CONTENT

INTRODUCTION

Interstitial cystitis, often known as IC, is an illness that affects the bladder and the urinary system. It is a chronic ailment that can be severe. In my capacity as a nutritionist, I am aware of the critical part that diet plays in the management of the symptoms associated with IC. In this all-encompassing book, we will dig into the complexities of IC, investigating what it is, its origins and triggers, and how dietary choices may have a big influence on the treatment of symptoms.

Understanding Interstitial Cystitis (IC)

Interstitial cystitis is a disorder that is defined by chronic discomfort or pain in the bladder and the surrounding pelvic region. At its core, this ailment is described as being complicated and involves several aspects. Formerly known as painful bladder syndrome, irritable bowel syndrome (IC) is an illness that is not well understood, and the specific etiology of the condition is still unknown. However, to effectively manage the problems that are associated with IC, it is essential for persons who are struggling with the illness to acquire a fundamental understanding of the disorder.

What is Interstitial Cystitis?

Chronic inflammation of the bladder wall is the initial indication of interstitial cystitis, which can cause a variety of symptoms that greatly impair a person's quality of life. Pelvic discomfort, urgency in urinating often, and a continuous sensation of bladder pressure are common symptoms. Because symptoms can differ in intensity from person to person, IC is a very personal experience.

Numerous ideas have been put out by medical professionals in the course of continuous research into the precise origin of IC. Some speculate that IC may develop as a result of a flaw in the bladder's protective lining that allows irritating compounds in urine to pass through the bladder wall. Some suggest an autoimmune component, in which the immune system of the body assaults and targets the bladder tissue by mistake. It's still unknown what exactly causes IC, despite these suggestions.

Living with IC may be difficult as the symptoms frequently mimic those of other urinary disorders, which can cause delayed or incorrect diagnoses. Patience, perseverance, and a multidisciplinary approach which may involve pharmacological interventions, lifestyle changes, and most importantly dietary modifications are necessary on the path to comprehending and controlling IC.

<h1 style="text-align:center">Causes and Triggers</h1>

To properly manage IC, it is imperative to identify its unique causes and triggers. Certain circumstances are known to worsen symptoms and lead to flare-ups, however, the underlying reason is still unknown.

Potential Causes:

- **Bladder Lining Defects:** Some people with IC may have flaws in the bladder's lining, which increases the likelihood of irritation and inflammation.

- **Autoimmune Factors:** One possible cause of IC is an autoimmune reaction, in which the immune system of the body unintentionally attacks and destroys the tissue of the bladder.

- **Genetic Predisposition:** Some people may be more genetically inclined to get IC than others. Bladder Lining Defects: Some people with IC may have flaws in the bladder's lining, which increases the likelihood of irritation and inflammation.

- **Autoimmune Factors:** One possible cause of IC is an autoimmune reaction, in which the immune system of the body unintentionally attacks and destroys the tissue of the bladder.
- **Genetic Predisposition:** Some people may be more genetically inclined to get IC than others.

Triggers:

- Dietary Triggers: Several meals and drinks have been shown to often cause symptoms of IC. Acidic foods, coffee, artificial sweeteners, spicy meals, and alcohol are a few examples of them.

- Stress and Emotional Factors: Anxiety and emotional stress can make IC symptoms worse, emphasizing how closely the mind and body are linked in the management of this illness.

- Allergies and urinary tract infections: For certain people, allergies and urinary tract infections can cause IC symptoms.

Developing a comprehensive strategy for treating IC requires an understanding of how these causes and triggers interact with one another. Medication adjustments are important for symptom relief and improving general health, even if they may not treat every facet of the illness.

Managing Symptoms through Diet

I understand the tremendous influence food decisions may have on controlling IC symptoms because I work as a dietician. Identifying and removing possible trigger foods while emphasizing healthy, anti-inflammatory choices are key components of creating an IC-friendly diet. Keeping the following points in mind while using food to control symptoms:

- IC-Friendly Meals: It's important to focus on foods that are less prone to cause bladder irritation. Lean meats, whole grains, and low-acid fruits and vegetables are examples of this. Including them in a well-balanced diet can supply necessary nutrients without producing side effects.

- Foods to Avoid: For those with IC, avoiding recognized triggers is essential. This might entail cutting back on or giving up acidic foods, coffee, alcohol, and artificial sweeteners. Identifying personal triggers can be greatly aided by maintaining a food diary.

- Hydration: People with IC need to make sure they are getting enough water. Drinking extra water may seem contradictory while experiencing urinary problems, but being properly hydrated promotes general health and helps remove irritants from the bladder.

- Nutritional Supplements: Some supplements, such as quercetin and omega-3 fatty acids, have demonstrated the potential to lower inflammation and ease the symptoms of IC. But before adding supplements to the diet, it's imperative to speak with a medical expert.

We will go further into various nutritional approaches in this extensive book, including helpful hints, recipes, and meal plans customized for people with IC. Those with Interstitial Cystitis can take proactive measures to manage their symptoms and enhance their overall quality of life by learning the subtleties of the illness and embracing a mindful approach to diet.

CHAPTER 1: BASICS OF INTERSTITIAL CYSTITIS DIET

Interstitial cystitis (IC) is a condition that frequently requires a sophisticated and thorough approach to the decisions that are made about one's diet. A substantial influence on the symptoms that are linked with this ailment can be exerted by the meals that we consume. In this chapter, we will discuss the fundamentals of an IC-friendly diet, including an overview of appropriate foods, foods that should be avoided, the significance of being hydrated, and ideas for meal planning that are both practical and useful.

Overview of IC-Friendly Foods

To adopt a diet that is favorable to individuals with IC, it is important to prioritize foods that are less likely to irritate the bladder and make symptoms worse. Even though the sensitivities of different people might vary, there are broad recommendations that can be used as a basis for developing a diet that is both well-balanced and nourishing for those who have sensitivity to certain foods.

- Low-Acid Fruits and Vegetables: An important part of an IC-friendly diet is emphasizing fruits and vegetables that are low in acidity. Nutrient-dense foods like cucumbers, pears, and blueberries can satisfy your need for vitamins and minerals without irritating your skin.

- Lean Proteins: People with IC may benefit from including lean proteins in their diet, such as fish, chicken, and tofu. These protein sources offer vital amino acids for general health and are less prone to cause inflammation.

- Whole Grains: Choosing whole grains helps increase dietary fiber content without adding too much acidity. Examples of these grains are brown rice, quinoa, and oats. In addition to being beneficial for general health, fiber is necessary for digestive health.

- Dairy substitutes: Conventional dairy products might irritate a lot of people with IC. Discovering lactose-free or almond milk alternatives to dairy enables the enjoyment of creamy textures without aggravating symptoms.

- Herbs and Spices: When adding flavor to IC-friendly foods, it's important to use herbs and spices that are well-tolerated. Fresh herbs, such as dill, parsley, and basil, can improve the flavor of food without becoming uncomfortable.

- Drinks Without Citrus: Selecting drinks without citrus, such as water, herbal teas, and certain non-acidic fruit juices, promotes hydration without adding any possible triggers. Maintaining enough hydration is crucial for eliminating irritants from the bladder.

Foods to Avoid

One of the most important aspects of controlling interstitial cystitis is recognizing and avoiding trigger foods. Although each person's triggers are unique, several common offenders have been found. People who have IC must be extremely watchful of what they eat and note how different foods affect their symptoms. The following dietary groups should be avoided:

- Acidic Foods: It is well known that citrus fruits, tomatoes, and vinegar-containing items are acidic and can irritate the lining of the bladder. To avoid flare-ups, people with IC may want to restrict or avoid certain foods.

- Coffee: Caffeine is a well-known irritant of the bladder that can make symptoms of IC worse. Chocolate, coffee, tea, and certain drinks should be drunk in moderation or not at all.

- Spicy Foods: For people with IC, spices like spicy sauce and chili peppers might be troublesome. It is best to go with gentler options as they might exacerbate symptoms and cause inflammation.

- Artificial Sweeteners: There have been reports that some artificial sweeteners, including those that include saccharin, aspartame, and sucralose, might cause symptoms of IC. It could be safer to go with natural sweeteners like honey or maple syrup.

- Alcohol: Alcohol can irritate the bladder and cause inflammation, particularly beer and wine. For those with IC, limiting alcohol use or selecting non-alcoholic substitutes may be helpful.

- Prepared and Hot Foods: Treat processed foods rich in chemicals and preservatives as well as hot snacks with prudence. These could have unidentified factors that exacerbate symptoms.

People with IC are better equipped to make decisions that are in line with their unique sensitivities when they are aware of these possible trigger foods. It's important to remember that different meals might have different effects, and maintaining a food journal can be a useful tool for figuring out what triggers you personally.

Importance of Hydration

Sufficient hydration is essential for good health in general and much more so for those who have Interstitial Cystitis. Although drinking extra fluids can seem paradoxical for treating urinary problems, maintaining proper hydration is crucial for several reasons:

Flushing Irritants: Maintaining a healthy urinary system involves flushing irritants and toxins from the bladder with enough fluids. In general, the bladder lining is less irritated by diluted urine.

Avoiding Concentrated Urine: The symptoms of IC may worsen if there is a dehydration-related increase in concentrated urine. Urine is more likely to be sufficiently diluted when proper hydration levels are maintained, which lowers the chance of discomfort.

Supporting General Health: Drinking enough water has a positive influence on several body processes, such as digestion, circulation, and temperature control. Maintaining adequate hydration is beneficial to the health of people with IC.

In order to maximize hydration and minimize possible triggers, people with IC may want to consider drinking non-citrus drinks including water, herbal teas, and some fruit juices. Urine color may be used as a straightforward measure of one's level of hydration; a pale yellow tint indicates sufficient hydration.

Tips for Meal Planning with IC

Careful meal planning is necessary for the effective dietary management of interstitial cystitis. To build a well-balanced and IC-friendly food plan, take into account the following advice:

- Diversify Your Plate: Make sure your meals contain nutritious grains, lean proteins, and a range of low-acid fruits and vegetables. A wide variety of nutrients is guaranteed when you diversify your plate and don't rely too much on foods that may cause triggers.

- Try Different Components: To make tasty recipes without sacrificing flavor, experiment with different ingredients and substitutes. For instance, consider substituting dairy products for creamy textures or using herbs and spices in place of acidic condiments.

- Practice Portion Control: Be mindful of serving sizes to prevent overindulging, which can strain the bladder more. For some people, eating smaller, more frequent meals throughout the day may be advantageous.

- Keep a Food Journal: Keep a food journal to monitor your dietary decisions and symptoms. This can aid in the identification of trends and the identification of certain trigger meals, enabling better-informed decision-making.

- It's Important to Practice Preparation: Try out various cooking techniques. Cooking techniques including grilling, steaming, and baking are frequently less taxing on the digestive tract than high-heat or frying.

- Keep Up: Remain up to date on the latest findings and available information regarding diets that are IC-friendly. Dietary guidelines might change over time, so it's important to remain up to date on the newest findings to make sure your meal plan reflects the most recent thinking.

CHAPTER 2: CREATING AN IC-FRIENDLY KITCHEN

In the process of managing interstitial cystitis (IC) with food, the setting in which meals are prepared is an important factor to consider. The creation of a kitchen that is suitable for individuals with intellectual disabilities requires careful planning, the strategic stocking of pantry essentials, and the guaranteeing of the availability of important kitchen instruments. Learning how to read food labels is also an important ability to acquire since it enables one to make well-informed decisions that follow the dietary rules of the International Community.

Stocking IC-Friendly Pantry Staples

A well-stocked pantry is the starting point for making meals that are both IC-friendly and healthy. Here's how to fill your cupboard with essentials that won't as frequently cause symptoms of IC:

- Whole Grains: Choose whole grains like oats, brown rice, and quinoa. These grains offer nutrients and vital fiber without the acidity of processed grains.

- Low-Acid Canned Goods: Keep your pantry stocked with low-acid canned foods such as lentils, chickpeas, and beans. These high-protein choices don't irritate the bladder and may be used as a foundation for many other recipes.

- Non-Citrus Vinegars: Although conventional vinegar can be acidic, there are non-citrus kinds of vinegar that could be easier to handle, such as apple cider vinegar or rice vinegar. Use them sparingly to add taste without aggravating symptoms.

- Herbs and Spices: Compile a selection of flavor-enhancing herbs and spices that won't irritate skin. Think about herbs like dill, thyme, basil, and oregano. Taste-testing different mixtures helps improve the flavor of IC-friendly recipes.

- IC-Friendly Oils: Opt for oils like avocado or olive oil that are easy on the digestive tract. These can be added to food or used as salad dressings.

- Low-Acid Sweeteners: Use low-acid sweeteners, such as honey or maple syrup, in place of conventional sweeteners. You may add sweetness with these natural sweeteners without causing discomfort to your bladder.

- Non-Dairy Substitutes: Examine non-dairy substitutes such as almond, coconut, or oat milk. These can be used in place of regular dairy products in baking and cooking, which may exacerbate IC symptoms.

- Low-Acid Grains and Pasta: Serve pasta prepared from substitute flours, like rice or chickpea flour, or low-acid grains, like quinoa. These choices provide you flexibility while preparing meals that are IC-friendly.

Keeping your pantry well-stocked with these IC-friendly essentials can help you prepare meals that meet your dietary requirements.

Essential Kitchen Tools for IC-Friendly Cooking

Cooking for someone with cancer may be more efficient and pleasurable if you have the proper kitchen utensils. The following is a list of necessary kitchen tools to think about:

- Blender or food processor: These appliances are great for making creamy soups, sauces, and purees without the use of harsh or corrosive substances.

- Vegetable Spiralizer: This inventive and low-acid substitute for traditional pasta lets you spiralize veggies into forms resembling noodles.

- Investing in non-stick cookware can help reduce the amount of cooking oil that is used excessively. This facilitates cooking and sautéing meals without adding any possible irritants.

- Herb Keeper: By preserving the freshness of herbs, a herb keeper makes sure that you always have savory alternatives available to add flavor to food.

- Citrus Squeezer with Filter: If you can only handle a limited amount of citrus, this citrus squeezer with filter can help you get juice free of pulp and seeds.

- Meal Planning App or Food Diary: Using a meal planning app or keeping a food diary might help you keep track of your dietary choices, symptoms, and well-received meals. When creating IC-friendly meal plans and detecting trigger foods, this tool can be quite helpful.

- Low-Acid Cutting Boards: You may want to use cutting boards made of high-density polyethylene or bamboo, which are both easily cleaned and less prone to contain bacteria.

- IC-Friendly Utensils: Choose utensils composed of materials that won't contaminate food with hazardous compounds. A suitable substitutes for plastic cutlery are silicone or stainless steel.

- Blender or food processor: These appliances are great for making creamy soups, sauces, and purees without the use of harsh or corrosive substances.

Keeping these basic kitchen utensils on hand makes cooking more convenient and makes it easier to prepare IC-friendly meals.

Reading Food Labels for IC

Getting around the grocery store aisles might be difficult, particularly if you have Interstitial Cystitis. Understanding food labels is an essential ability that enables people to make wise decisions and steer clear of any triggers. When reading food labels for IC, keep the following points in mind:

- Look for Acidic Ingredients: Peruse the ingredient list and look for acidic ingredients like vinegar, citrus, or tomatoes. If certain substances are known to trigger your symptoms, stay away from items containing them.

- Watch Out for Artificial Additives: Preservatives, colorings, and artificial additives can irritate people with IC. When it's feasible, pick entire, unadulterated meals and goods with little additives.

- Keep an eye on the salt content: Processed meals with high sodium content might aggravate IC symptoms by causing inflammation. To limit salt intake, choose low-sodium substitutes or make meals with fresh ingredients.

- Determine Potential Allergens: Food allergies or sensitivities may also exist in certain IC patients. Keep an eye out for any allergies on food labels and make appropriate substitutions.

- Beware of Hidden Sugars: Consuming too much sugar might exacerbate inflammation. In ingredient lists, look for hidden sugars, which might be listed under numerous names like fructose, sucrose, or high fructose corn syrup.

- Recognize Portion Sizes: Take note of the serving sizes that are shown on food labels. A product may appear to have a low concentration of a certain irritant at times, yet the serving size may be less than what is usually consumed.

- Think About Organic Options: Choosing organic items might help some people with IC feel less exposed to chemicals and pesticides that could aggravate their symptoms.

- Utilize Applications and Web Resources: You can expeditiously analyze food labels with the help of smartphone apps and online resources. Some applications, which let you scan barcodes for instant information, are made especially to support those with dietary restrictions.

Grocery shopping becomes a more efficient and knowledgeable procedure as you get better at reading food labels. With time, you'll become adept at identifying the goods that fit within your IC-friendly diet, which will simplify the overall treatment of interstitial cystitis.

CHAPTER 3: BREAKFAST RECIPES

Breakfast is frequently regarded as the most important meal of the day, and for those who suffer from interstitial cystitis (IC), it is of the utmost importance to prepare a breakfast that is in proper alignment with their nutritional requirements. A wide range of breakfast foods that are suitable for individuals with IC is discussed in this chapter. These recipes include grain-free pancakes and waffles, as well as breakfast bowls that are both delicious and refreshing.

IC-Friendly Smoothies

Smoothies are a flexible and practical breakfast choice that lets you include healthy components without worrying about triggers. The following smoothie recipes are IC-friendly and put the health of your bladder first:

1. Berry Bliss Smoothie:

Ingredients:

- One cup of blueberries (low-acid).
- Sliced strawberries, half a cup.
- 1 ripe banana.
- Almond milk in one cup (or non-dairy alternative).
- One spoonful of honey (optional, for sweetness).
- Cubes of ice.

Instructions:

1. Mix all of the ingredients until they are completely smooth.
2. If you want the sweetness to be adjusted, honey can be used.
3. Enjoy this smoothie that is loaded with antioxidants by pouring it into a glass.

2. Creamy Tropical Delight:

Ingredients:

- Half a cup of chunky pineapple
- Mango pieces in a half-cup
- Half a ripe avocado
- One cup of coconut water
- One-third cup of chia seeds
- Cubes of ice

Instructions:

1. Mix each item in a blender until smooth.
2. To get the right consistency, add extra coconut water.

3. For extra texture and nutritional value, top with chia seeds.

3. Green Goddess Smoothie:

Ingredients:

- 1 cup of spinach leaves.
- 1/2 cucumber, peeled and sliced.
- 1/2 green apple, cored and cut.
- Juiced half a lemon.
- One cup of coconut water or water.
- Cubes of ice.

Instructions:

1. Mix every item until it's smooth.
2. You can use water or coconut water to adjust the consistency.
3. Juice from a lemon squeezed for a cool kick.

4. Rich in vitamins, minerals, and antioxidants, these IC-friendly smoothies stay away from traditional triggers like citrus and acidic fruits.

Low-Acid Breakfast Bowls

Breakfast bowls offer a customizable and satisfying way to start the day. By selecting low-acid fruits, incorporating grains mindfully, and adding protein-rich elements, you can create a breakfast bowl that caters to IC dietary guidelines.

1. Quinoa Breakfast Bowl:

Ingredients:

- Half a cup of cooked quinoa
- Half a cup of blueberries (low-acid)
- Half a banana, sliced
- One spoonful of butter made with almonds
- One spoonful of chia seeds
- A spritz of almond milk

Instructions:

1. Transfer the cooked quinoa to a bowl.

2. Top with blueberries, banana slices, and almond butter.

3. Incorporate chia seeds and a small amount of almond milk.

4. Mix and savor this breakfast dish full of protein.

2. Greek Yogurt Parfait:

Ingredients:

- One cup of Greek yogurt, plain
- 1/2 cup of peach dice (low-acid).
- 1/4 cup of granola (low-acid, with no added triggers).
- One spoonful of honey
- One tablespoon of finely chopped almonds

Instructions:

1. Arrange Greek yogurt slices in a dish.
2. Add granola and sliced peaches.

3. After adding a honey drizzle, top with chopped almonds.
4. Make several layers for a tasty and aesthetically pleasing parfait.

3. Chia Seed Pudding Bowl:

Ingredients:

- Two tsp of chia seeds
- Half a cup of almond milk
- One-half tsp vanilla extract
- Half a cup of raspberries (low-acid).
- One tablespoon of coconut shreds.

Instructions:

1. In a dish, combine almond milk, vanilla essence, and chia seeds.
2. Put in the fridge for several hours or perhaps overnight to get a pudding-like consistency.

3. Before serving, sprinkle shredded coconut and raspberries over top.

4. These ideas for breakfast bowls emphasize utilizing foods that are easy on the bladder while combining a variety of textures and flavors.

Grain-Free Pancakes and Waffles

Pancakes and waffles can still be served to folks who are looking for grain-free choices without making them feel like IC symptoms. You may have a tasty, bladder-friendly breakfast by using alternate flours and choosing your toppings wisely.

1. Almond Flour Pancakes:

Ingredients:

- A cup of almond flour.
- 2 eggs.
- Half a cup of almond milk.
- 1 tablespoon of oil from coconut.
- 1/2 teaspoon of baking powder.
- Half a teaspoon of vanilla extract.

Instructions:

1. Almond flour, eggs, almond milk, baking powder, coconut oil, and vanilla extract should all be combined in a bowl.
2. To create pancakes, preheat a nonstick pan and ladle batter onto it.
3. Cook until bubbles appear, then turn and continue cooking the other side.
4. Serve with sliced strawberries or other low-acid fruits.

2. Coconut Flour Waffles:

Ingredients:

- Half a cup of coconut flour
- Four eggs
- half a cup of coconut milk
- Two teaspoons of coconut oil melted
- One-half tsp baking soda
- Half a teaspoon of extract from vanilla

Instructions:

1. Mix the coconut flour, eggs, milk, baking soda, melted coconut oil, and vanilla essence in a bowl.
2. Before adding batter, preheat your waffle machine.
3. Cook till crisp and golden brown.
4. Place low-acid fruits on top and pour maple syrup over them.

3. Banana-Oat Blender Pancakes:

Ingredients:

- Two fully ripe bananas
- Two eggs
- Half a cup of rolled oats
- One-half tsp baking powder
- Half a teaspoon of extract from vanilla
- A dash of salt

Instructions:

Ripe bananas, eggs, rolled oats, baking powder, vanilla essence, and a little teaspoon of salt should all be combined in a blender.

Process till smooth.

Use a nonstick pan or griddle to cook pancakes.

Serve with low-acid fruit and a dollop of Greek yogurt.

These tasty and texture-rich grain-free pancake and waffle recipes satisfy anyone on an IC-friendly diet.

CHAPTER 4: LUNCH AND DINNER RECIPES

Those who have interstitial cystitis have the opportunity to enjoy scrumptious and fulfilling meals while following the dietary constraints that are associated with the condition (IC). In this chapter, we will discuss salads that are ideal for those with IC and are high in protein, soups that are cozy and do not include trigger items, and main course alternatives that are appropriate for both lunch and supper.

Protein-Rich IC-Friendly Salads

Salads are a flexible base from which to create nutrient-dense meals that meet the dietary criteria for those with IC. You may have satisfying salads that improve your overall health by adding lean meats, low-acid veggies, and dressings that are kind to your bladder.

1. Grilled Chicken and Berry Salad:

Ingredients:
- Sliced chicken breast from the grill.
- mixed greens for salad.
- Blueberries.
- strawberries cut into slices.
- chopped avocado
- Grapefruit vinaigrette (made with low-acid vinegar).

Instructions:

1. On a platter, arrange mixed salad greens.

2. Add chopped avocado, sliced strawberries, blueberries, and grilled chicken on top.

3. Add a homemade balsamic vinaigrette and drizzle.

4. Enjoy this salad, which is full of nutrition and refreshing, by tossing gently.

2. Quinoa and Veggie Bowl with Shrimp:

Ingredients:

- Cherry tomatoes, halved

- Cucumber, diced

- Cooked quinoa

- Feta cheese (optional)

- Lemon-tahini dressing

- Grilled shrimp

- Red bell pepper, sliced

Instructions:

- In a bowl, mix the quinoa, red bell pepper, cucumber, cherry tomatoes, and grilled shrimp.
- If preferred, top with feta cheese.
- Pour over some lemon-tahini dressing to create a tasty, high-protein dish.

3. Tofu and Asian-Inspired Salad:

Ingredients:

- Edamame beans
- Sesame seeds
- Cubed tofu, sautéed or baked
- Ginger-soy dressing
- Mixed greens
- Shredded carrots

Instructions:

1. Put mixed greens together on a platter.

2. Add the edamame beans, shredded carrots, and tofu, either baked or sautéed.

3. Add sesame seeds on the top.

4. Pour over ginger-soy dressing for a taste of Asia.

5. These salads are high in protein and offer you a good mix of nutrients without making you feel like you have IC.

Comforting Soups without Trigger Ingredients

Warm and soothing soups are a great choice for lunch or dinner, especially when made with ingredients that are favorable to IC. Sleek meats, low-acid veggies, and steering clear of frequent triggers can allow you to savor a cup of soup that relieves without increasing symptoms.

1. Butternut Squash and Carrot Soup:

Ingredients:

- Onion, diced
- Vegetable broth
- Coconut milk
- Carrots, chopped
- Ginger, minced
- Cumin, ground
- Salt and pepper to taste

- Butternut squash, peeled and diced

Instructions:

1. Saute onion in a saucepan till it becomes transparent.
2. Add the ground cumin, carrots, cubed butternut squash, and ginger.
3. After adding the vegetable broth, boil the veggies until they are soft.
4. After blending until smooth, stir in the coconut milk.
5. To taste, add salt and pepper for seasoning.

2. Chicken and Rice Soup:

Ingredients:

- Carrots, sliced
- Celery, diced

- Chicken broth
- Cooked chicken breast, shredded
- Brown rice, cooked
- Parsley, chopped
- Lemon juice
- Salt and pepper to taste

Instructions:

1. Shredded chicken, cooked brown rice, chopped celery, carrots, and chicken broth should all be combined in a saucepan.
2. Simmer the veggies until they are soft.
3. Add the lemon juice and chopped parsley and stir.
4. To taste, add salt and pepper for seasoning.

3. Lentil and Vegetable Soup:

Ingredients:

- Onion, diced
- Carrots, diced
- Celery, diced
- Green lentils, rinsed
- Vegetable broth
- Spinach leaves
- Italian seasoning
- Tomatoes, diced (low-acid variety)
- Salt and pepper to taste

Instructions:

1. The diced onion should be sautéed till tender in a saucepan.
2. Add the chopped tomatoes, carrots, and celery along with the green lentils and vegetable broth.

3. Lentils should be cooked fully after simmering.

4. Add the spinach leaves, Italian seasoning, and salt & pepper to taste.

5. These hearty soups are perfect for lunch or dinner since they are warm and nourishing without going beyond IC dietary requirements.

Main Course Options for Lunch and Dinner

Main dishes play a vital part in lunch and supper, and by using IC-friendly components, you may make delectable and fulfilling meals. These are the main course alternatives that are tailored to the needs of bladder health.

1. Baked Salmon with Dill Sauce:

Ingredients:

- Salmon fillets
- Lemon juice
- Garlic, minced
- Dill, chopped
- Greek yogurt (low-fat)
- Salt and pepper to taste

Instructions:

1. Place the salmon fillets on a baking tray and preheat the oven.
2. Add a lemon juice drizzle and chopped dill on top.
3. Bake the fish until it is well done.
4. Combine Greek yogurt, finely chopped garlic, and salt & pepper in a bowl.
5. Serve the dill sauce beside the cooked fish.

2. Turkey and Vegetable Stir-Fry:

Ingredients:

- Ground turkey
- Low-sodium soy sauce
- Ginger, minced
- Garlic, minced
- Sesame oil
- Broccoli florets
- Bell peppers, sliced

- Zucchini, sliced
- Brown rice (optional)

Instructions:

1. Cook the ground turkey until browned in a wok or pan.
2. Add the zucchini, broccoli florets, and bell peppers in slices.
3. Add minced garlic and ginger and stir.
4. Drizzle the stir-fry with sesame oil and reduced-sodium soy sauce.
5. If preferred, serve over brown rice.

3. Eggplant and Chickpea Curry:

Ingredients:

- Turmeric
- Cilantro, chopped
- Basmati rice
- Eggplant, diced

- Chickpeas, cooked
- Onion, diced
- Tomatoes, diced (low-acid variety)
- Coconut milk
- Curry powder

Instructions:

1. Diced onion should be cooked in a pan until tender.
2. Add the chopped tomatoes, cooked chickpeas, curry powder, turmeric, and coconut milk.
3. Cook until the eggplant becomes soft.
4. After adding some chopped cilantro, serve the dish over basmati rice.

These main course alternatives provide a range of flavors and textures while keeping to IC dietary rules. To fit your tastes, feel free to experiment with different proteins, veggies, and seasonings.

CHAPTER 5: SNACKS AND APPETIZERS

In between meals, snacks, and appetizers are important for sustaining energy levels and sating appetites. Making dietary guideline-compliant snack choices is crucial for those with Interstitial Cystitis (IC). This chapter will include finger foods that are appropriate for social events, healthy snack alternatives, and dips and spreads that are IC-friendly.

Nutritious Snack Ideas

Choosing nutrient-dense meals for your body during a snack will help you stay away from things that can aggravate your IC symptoms. The following healthy snack suggestions are made with the health of your bladder in mind:

1. Greek Yogurt Parfait:

Ingredients:

- Almond slices
- Honey
- Plain Greek yogurt
- Low-acid berries (e.g., blueberries, raspberries)

Instructions:

1. Arrange low-acid fruit on top of Greek yogurt in a glass or dish.
2. In between layers, scatter almond pieces.

3. Pour some honey over it to make it sweeter.

2. Hummus and Veggie Sticks:

Ingredients:

- Cucumber slices
- Bell pepper strips
- Hummus (low-acid or homemade)
- Carrot sticks

Instructions:

Dip bell pepper strips, cucumber slices, and carrot sticks into hummus.

Hummus provides a protein-rich and tasty snack, while veggies provide crunch and moisture.

3. Rice Cake with Avocado and Cherry Tomatoes:

Ingredients:

- Brown rice cakes
- Sprinkle of salt and pepper
- Avocado, mashed
- Cherry tomatoes, halved

Instructions:

1. Mash some avocado and top some brown rice cakes with it.
2. Arrange the halved cherry tomatoes on top.
3. For an easy and filling snack, just sprinkle with salt & pepper.

4. Cottage Cheese with Pineapple:

Ingredients:

- Low-fat cottage cheese
- Pineapple chunks

Instructions:

1. Toss together pieces of pineapple and low-fat cottage cheese.
2. Pineapple brings a hint of sweetness while cottage cheese gives protein.

5. Almond Butter and Banana Slices:

Ingredients:

- Almond butter
- Banana, sliced

Instructions:

1. Toast the banana slices with almond butter.

2. This snack has natural sweetness, protein, and good fats.

3. These wholesome snack suggestions include a balance of macronutrients and are readily adaptable to individual dietary requirements and tastes.

IC-Friendly Dips and Spreads

Not only are dips and spreads flexible, but they also can enhance the enjoyment of appetizers and snacks. Here are some possibilities that are suitable for those with IC and make use of fresh, low-acid ingredients:

1. Guacamole:

Ingredients:

- Lime juice
- Ripe avocados, mashed
- Cilantro, chopped
- Salt and pepper to taste
- Diced tomatoes (low-acid variety)
- Red onion, finely chopped

Instructions:

1. Put the mashed avocados, diced tomatoes, chopped red onion, and chopped cilantro into a bowl and mix them.

2. The mixture should be seasoned with salt and pepper, and lime juice should be squeezed over it.

3. Mix thoroughly, and serve with tortilla chips or vegetable sticks that have a low acid content.

2. Tzatziki:

Ingredients:

- Fresh dill, chopped
- Garlic, minced
- Greek yogurt
- Cucumber, finely diced
- Lemon juice
- Salt and pepper to taste

Instructions:

1. Greek yogurt, minced garlic, chopped fresh dill, sliced cucumber, and lemon juice should all be combined in a dish.

2. Add pepper and salt for seasoning.

3. Whole-grain pita or cucumber slices go nicely with tzatziki.

3. Roasted Red Pepper Hummus:

Ingredients:

- Garlic, minced

- Lemon juice

- Olive oil

- Chickpeas, drained and rinsed

- Roasted red peppers (from a jar, low-acid)

- Tahini

- Salt and cumin to taste

Instructions:

1. Puree the chickpeas, tahini, roasted red peppers, minced garlic, lemon juice, olive oil, salt, and cumin in a food processor until smooth.

2. Accompany with whole-grain crackers or veggie sticks.

4. Baba Ganoush:

Ingredients:

- Lemon juice
- Olive oil
- Eggplant
- Tahini
- Garlic, minced
- Salt and pepper to taste

Instructions:

1. Grilled or roasted eggplant is tender.
2. After peeling the skin, puree the meat with olive oil, lemon juice, chopped garlic, tahini, salt, and pepper.

3. Savor it with whole-grain pita or cucumber slices.

These IC-acceptable spreads and dips offer a taste explosion that complies with dietary guidelines.

Finger Foods for Social Gatherings

Sharing finger snacks is a common social gathering activity, and you may still engage in social events while following IC dietary rules. Here are some finger snack suggestions that work well for parties:

1. Caprese Skewers:

Ingredients:

- Basil leaves
- Balsamic glaze
- Cherry tomatoes (low-acid variety)
- Fresh mozzarella balls

Instructions:

1. Put a cherry tomato, a ball of fresh mozzarella, and a leaf of basil on a little skewer.

2. Place on a serving dish and pour balsamic glaze over.

2. Smoked Salmon Cucumber Bites:

Ingredients:

- Cream cheese (optional)
- Fresh dill
- English cucumber, sliced
- Smoked salmon

Instructions:

1. Add some smoked salmon to the cucumber slices.
2. Add a little dollop of cream cheese, if desired.
3. Place some fresh dill on top.

3. Stuffed Mini Peppers:

Ingredients:

- Goat cheese
- Chopped chives
- Mini sweet peppers, halved and seeds removed
- Walnuts, chopped

Instructions:

1. Combine chopped chives with goat cheese.
2. Stuff the goat cheese mixture into the little pepper halves.
3. Add chopped walnuts to the top.

4. Spinach and Feta Phyllo Triangles:

Ingredients:

- Phyllo dough sheets
- Olive oil
- Frozen spinach, thawed and drained
- Feta cheese, crumbled

Instructions:

1. Combine crumbled feta with thawed spinach.
2. Cut phyllo dough sheets into squares.
3. In the middle of each square, place a tablespoon of the spinach and feta mixture.
4. After folding into triangles, coat with olive oil.
5. Cook till the color turns golden.

5. Grilled Shrimp Skewers:

Ingredients:

- Garlic, minced

- Lemon zest

- Shrimp, peeled and deveined

- Olive oil

- Paprika

- Salt and pepper to taste

Instructions:

1. Shrimp should be marinated in olive oil, salt, pepper, paprika, lemon zest, and chopped garlic.

2. After skewering the shrimp, simmer them until done.

3. Garnish with a freshly squeezed lemon.

These finger meals are perfect for social occasions where dietary restrictions may differ since they are visually appealing and satisfy a variety of palates.

CHAPTER 6: DESSERTS AND SWEET TREATS

There are methods for people who have interstitial cystitis (IC) to experience the delights of sweets and sweet snacks while still sticking to dietary requirements. Indulging in these kinds of delicacies may be a joyful part of life. In this chapter, we will discuss recipes for low-acid desserts, fruit alternatives to fulfill sweet desires, and recipes for baked products that are suitable for those with IC and that satisfy without causing complications.

Low-Acid Dessert Recipes

Individuals who are controlling IC should prioritize the creation of desserts that contain low-acid components. In these recipes, the emphasis is placed on using foods that are easy on the bladder while yet providing a satisfying level of sweetness and flavor.

1. Vanilla Rice Pudding:

Ingredients:

- Arborio rice
- Vanilla extract
- Maple syrup
- Almond milk (or non-dairy alternative)
- Cinnamon

Instructions:

1. In almond milk, cook Arborio rice until it's creamy.

2. Add the vanilla essence and maple syrup to taste.

3. Before serving, give it a cinnamon sprinkle.

2. Coconut and Berry Popsicles:

Ingredients:

- Coconut milk
- Agave syrup or honey
- Mixed berries (low-acid varieties)

Instructions:

1. Mix mixed berries with coconut milk and add honey or agave syrup for sweetness.

2. Fill the molds with the mixture, then freeze for solidification.

3. Savor a low-acid, refreshing pleasure.

3. Baked Apples with Cinnamon:

Ingredients:

- Cinnamon
- Brown sugar (optional)
- Apples, cored and sliced
- Chopped nuts (optional)

Instructions:

1. Arrange the apple slices in a baking dish and preheat the oven.
2. If desired, dust with brown sugar and cinnamon.
3. Bake the apples until they are soft.
4. For extra crunch, sprinkle chopped nuts on top.

4. Chia Seed and Mango Pudding:

Ingredients:

- Chia seeds
- Ripe mango, diced
- Agave syrup or honey
- Almond milk (or non-dairy alternative)

Instructions:

1. Blend almond milk and chia seeds, then set aside until a pudding-like consistency develops.
2. Add chopped mango to the layer and use honey or agave syrup for sweetness.
3. Chill before serving.
4. For persons with IC, these low-acid dessert dishes provide a variety of flavors and textures, making them pleasant alternatives.

Fruit Alternatives for Sweet Cravings

Discovering fruit alternatives that are lower in acidity can be a game-changer for those who suffer from intellectual disability (IC). Here are some sweet alternatives to fruits that are commonly consumed:

1. Baked Pears with Caramel Sauce:

Ingredients:

- Coconut oil
- Cinnamon
- Pears, halved and cored
- Coconut sugar

Instructions:

1. Arrange the pear halves in a baking tray and preheat the oven.
2. Add cinnamon and coconut sugar over top.
3. Pour over some melted coconut oil.

4. Bake the pears until they become soft and caramelized.

2. Grilled Peaches with Honey:

Ingredients:

- Honey
- Peaches, halved and pitted
- Fresh mint leaves (optional)

Instructions:

1. Halve the peaches and set them on the preheated grill.
2. Grill the peaches until they get grill marks.
3. If preferred, garnish with fresh mint leaves and drizzle with honey.

3. Cinnamon-Roasted Plums:

Ingredients:

- Cinnamon
- Maple syrup
- Plums, halved and pitted

Instructions:

1. Put the halves of the plums in a baking dish and preheat the oven.
2. Drizzle with maple syrup and sprinkle with cinnamon.
3. Roast plums until they become tender and caramelized.

4. Banana Nice Cream:

Ingredients:

- Frozen sliced ripe bananas
- Almond milk (or non-dairy alternative)
- Extract from vanilla

Instructions:

1. Blend almond milk, vanilla essence, and frozen banana slices till smooth.

2. For a naturally sweet and creamy frozen dessert, serve right away.

3. With the range of textures and tastes offered by these fruit substitutes, people with IC may indulge in their sweet tooth without experiencing symptoms.

IC-Friendly Baked Goods

Baking may be a reassuring addition to a dessert repertoire, and if you choose ingredients that are suitable for those with inflammatory bowel disease (IC), you can still enjoy the pleasure of making your sweets. The following is a list of recipes for baked items that fulfill the requirements of the IC dietary guidelines:

1. Oat Flour Banana Bread:

Ingredients:

- Eggs
- Coconut oil
- Oat flour
- Ripe bananas, mashed
- Baking powder
- Cinnamon

Instructions:

1. Combine eggs, melted coconut oil, baking powder, cinnamon, and mashed bananas with oat flour.
2. Fill the loaf pan, and bake until the toothpick inserted into the center comes out clean.

2. Almond Flour Blueberry Muffins:

Ingredients:

- Maple syrup
- Baking soda
- Almond flour
- Eggs
- Blueberries (low-acid)
- Vanilla extract

Instructions:

1. Add eggs, blueberries, baking soda, maple syrup, and vanilla extract to the almond flour mixture.

2. Fill muffin cups with batter, then bake until golden.

3. Coconut Flour Chocolate Chip Cookies:

Ingredients:

- Coconut oil
- Eggs
- Maple syrup
- Coconut flour
- Chocolate chips (low-acid variety)
- Vanilla extract

Instructions:

1. Mix coconut flour with melted coconut oil, eggs, maple syrup, chocolate chips, and vanilla essence.
2. Place on a baking sheet, shape into cookies, and bake until the edges are brown.

4. Pumpkin Spice Muffins:

Ingredients:

- Eggs
- Coconut oil
- Pumpkin spice
- Canned pumpkin
- Almond flour
- Baking powder

Instructions:

Almond flour, eggs, melted coconut oil, pumpkin spice, and baking powder should all be combined with canned pumpkin.

Stuff muffin tins full, then bake for the toothpick to come out clean.

You may still enjoy classic delights without compromising bladder health thanks to these IC-friendly baked products.

CHAPTER 7: BEVERAGES

Beverages are a crucial component of our day-to-day lives, and it is essential for people who are managing interstitial cystitis (IC) to choose beverages that are mild on the bladder. In this chapter, we will discuss hydration beverages that are suitable for individuals with irritable bowel syndrome (IC), herbal teas that provide relief from IC, and mocktail recipes that are made without the use of components that trigger IC.

Hydrating IC-Friendly Drinks

Maintaining proper hydration is essential for general health, and it is especially important for individuals who suffer from IC to select beverages that will not make their symptoms worse. The following are some alternatives that are suitable for IC that are hydrating:

1. Water Infusions:

Ingredients:

- Sliced cucumber
- Fresh mint leaves
- Filtered water
- Lemon slices (optional)

Instructions:

1. Pour purified water into a pitcher.
2. If tolerable, add cucumber slices, lemon slices, and fresh mint leaves.

3. Store it in the fridge to infuse it into a revitalizing beverage.

2. Coconut Water:

Ingredients:

- Pure coconut water

Instructions:

1. Select pure coconut water that hasn't had any flavors or sweets added.
2. Coconut water is not only hydrating but also delivers electrolytes.

3. Aloe Vera Juice:

Ingredients:

- Pure aloe vera juice

Instructions:

1. Select aloe vera juice that hasn't had any sugar or preservatives added.
2. Aloe vera is a moisturizing choice and is well-known for its calming qualities.

4. Peppermint Tea:

Ingredients:

- Hot water
- Peppermint tea bags

Instructions:

1. In boiling water, steep peppermint tea bags.
2. In addition to being cooling, peppermint tea has the potential to ease certain IC symptoms.

5. Sparkling Water with a Splash of Cranberry Juice:

Ingredients:

- Ice cubes
- Sparkling water
- Unsweetened cranberry juice

Instructions:

1. Mix sparkling water with a dash of unsweetened cranberry juice.

2. Add ice cubes for a fresh and hydrating beverage.

These hydrated, flavor-rich, IC-friendly beverages consider bladder health.

Herbal Teas for IC Relief

For people who are coping with the symptoms of IC, herbal teas can be a source of comfort and respite. These herbal teas are well-known for their calming effects, and they are as follows:

1. Chamomile Tea:

Ingredients:

- Hot water
- Chamomile tea bags

Instructions:

1. Use boiling water to steep chamomile tea packets.
2. It's well known that chamomile has anti-inflammatory and relaxing effects.

2. Marshmallow Root Tea:

Ingredients:

- Hot water
- Marshmallow root tea bags

Instructions:

1. Steep tea bags with marshmallow root in boiling water.
2. It is said that marshmallow root soothes the bladder.

3. Rooibos Tea:

Ingredients:

- Rooibos tea bags
- Hot water

Instructions:

1. Add boiling water to rooibos tea bags and steep.

2. Rooibos tea has a subtle sweetness and is devoid of caffeine.

4. Slippery Elm Bark Tea:

Ingredients:

- Hot water
- Slippery elm bark tea bags

Instructions:

1. Steep tea bags made of slippery elm bark in hot water.
2. Because of its high mucilage content, slippery elm bark has a calming effect.

5. Ginger Tea:

Ingredients:

- Hot water
- Fresh ginger, sliced

Instructions:

1. Soak newly cut ginger slices in warm water.
2. Because of its anti-inflammatory qualities, ginger could help with some IC symptoms.

These herbal teas offer possible relief as well as comfort and can be consumed warm or over ice.

Mocktail Recipes without Triggering Ingredients

The creation of mocktails that do not contain any components that might cause a reaction can be a great option for social gatherings or just when one is in the mood for a particular beverage. The following are some recipes for refreshing mocktails:

1. Cucumber Mint Mocktail:

Ingredients:

- Lime slices
- Ice cubes
- Sparkling water
- Sliced cucumber
- Fresh mint leaves

Instructions:

1. Sliced cucumber, fresh mint leaves, and lime slices should all be combined with sparkling water.
2. To make a drink that is chilly and revitalizing, add ice cubes.

2. Berry Basil Lemonade Mocktail:

Ingredients:

- Lemonade (unsweetened)
- Ice cubes
- Mixed berry puree (blueberries, raspberries, strawberries)
- Fresh basil leaves

Instructions:

1. Muddle some fresh basil leaves in a glass.
2. Pour in unsweetened lemonade and pureed mixed berries.
3. Mix well and pour onto ice.

3. Pineapple Coconut Cooler:

Ingredients:

- Coconut water
- Ice cubes
- Mint leaves
- Pineapple chunks
- Pineapple juice (unsweetened)

Instructions:

1. Blend pineapple juice without added sugar and coconut water.
2. Add pineapple pieces and mint leaves.
3. Serve over ice, shaking or stirring.

4. Lavender Lemon Sparkler:

Ingredients:

- Lavender-infused water (cooled)
- Sparkling water
- Ice cubes
- Fresh lemon juice
- Agave syrup (optional)

Instructions:

1. Add fresh lemon juice to water that has been steeped with lavender.
2. If desired, sweeten with agave syrup.
3. Top with sparkling water and ice cubes.

5. Minty Iced Green Tea:

Ingredients:

- Fresh mint leaves
- Honey (optional)
- Green tea bags
- Ice cubes

Instructions:

1. Use boiling water to steep green tea bags.
2. If desired, add some fresh mint leaves and sweeten with honey.
3. Allow it to cool, then serve over ice.

These mocktail recipes are good for people controlling IC since they provide a taste boost without utilizing frequent triggers.

CHAPTER 8: MEAL PLANNING AND BATCH COOKING

People who are managing interstitial cystitis can benefit greatly from the use of strong tools such as efficient meal planning and batch cooking (IC). It is possible to emphasize bladder-friendly foods while saving time and guaranteeing a diversified and delicious diet if you sensibly organize your meals. This chapter will cover a variety of topics, including tactics for weekly meal planning, the advantages of cooking in bulk for busy days, and advice for dining out with internet-connected people.

Weekly Meal Planning Strategies

To successfully plan meals, you must give careful consideration to your nutritional requirements, tastes, and schedule of activities. The following are some ideas that might help you plan your weekly meals:

1. Evaluate Your Timetable: Start by assessing the next week. Note any days that might affect your eating patterns, such as hectic schedules, social gatherings, or other circumstances.

2. Create a Menu: Arrange your weekly food plan based on your schedule. A variety of protein sources, low-acid veggies, and cereals or substitutes that are favorable to IC should be included.

3. Make a Detailed Shopping List: After you've decided on your meal, make a thorough shopping list. This makes it less likely that you will overlook important components and simplifies your grocery shopping process.

4. Embrace Variation: To guarantee a well-rounded nutritional intake, strive for variety in your meals. Vary your protein, veggie, and grain intake throughout the week.

5. Pre-Portion Items: You may save time during the week by preparing and portioning ingredients ahead of time. To make construction easier, chop veggies, marinade meats, or precooked grains.

6. Take Leftovers Into Account: Arrange meals with leftovers in mind. For instance, roast a whole chicken on Sunday to use all week long in stir-fries, salads, and wraps.

7. Be Adaptable: Give your strategy some leeway. Being flexible guarantees that you can continue to make IC-friendly decisions even if your plans alter since life is unpredictable.

8. Remain Hydrated: To promote bladder health, incorporate hydrating drinks into your schedule, such as herbal teas, coconut water, or water infusions.

You may simplify meal planning and make it a sustainable and controllable part of your routine by implementing these ideas.

Batch Cooking for Busy Days

During the process of batch cooking, bigger amounts of meals are prepared all at once to have ready-made alternatives available for days when time is restricted. Cooking in batches may be incorporated into your routine in the following ways:

1. Pick Recipes That Are Batch-Friendly:

Choose recipes, such as soups, stews, casseroles, or one-pan meals, that work well when cooked in large quantities.

2. Invest in Storage Containers: Get many various-sized storage containers. This enables you to divide out and store meals that are prepared in bulk for later use.

3. Set Aside Dedicated Time: Identify a particular day of the week to devote to batch cooking. This can take place on the weekends or on a day when you have more free time.

4. Make Use of Freezer-Friendly Foods: When creating recipes for bulk cooking, use ingredients that freeze well. Many soups, sauces, and cereals, for instance, may be frozen and reheated without losing their flavor.

5. Label and Date: Mark the contents and preparation date of each batch-cooked dish. This keeps food waste at bay and makes it easier to monitor freshness.

6. Mix & Match Components: Prepare ingredients in bulk that may be combined or separated to create a variety of dishes. For example, prepare a big pot of quinoa and serve it with various veggies and meats throughout the week.

7. Make a plan for busy days. In particular, prepare meals in bulk for days when your calendar is busy. The temptation to choose less bladder-friendly options is lessened when there is a ready-made, IC-friendly option available.

8. Accept Multitasking: Use your time wisely by engaging in many tasks at once. You may prepare the ingredients for another meal while the first one simmers on the burner.

In addition to saving time, batch cooking guarantees that you always have IC-friendly options on hand, encouraging consistency in your dietary decisions.

Tips for Dining Out with Interstitial Cystitis

A certain amount of planning and boldness is required to successfully navigate restaurant menus with IC. If you have interstitial cystitis, here are some suggestions for dining out:

1. Examine Menus in Ahead: A lot of eateries now post their menus online. Utilize this by looking over choices ahead of time to find selections that are acceptable to IC.

2. Express Your Needs: Don't be afraid to let the server know what foods you are allergic to when you go to the restaurant. Inquire about any adjustments or replacements of ingredients.

3. Select Baked or Grilled Options: Avoid fried foods by choosing baked or grilled alternatives. Vegetables and proteins that are grilled tend to be kinder to the bladder.

4. Request Dressings and Sauces on the Side: Ask for dressings and sauces on the side to help you limit the quantity of potentially irritating components. In this manner, you have the option to utilize them selectively or not at all.

5. Be Aware of Your Drinks: Consider the beverages you choose to consume. Choose IC-friendly beverages like water or herbal teas to remain hydrated without aggravating symptoms.

6. Ask About Substitutes of Ingredients: Do not be afraid to ask about substitutions of ingredients. A lot of eateries are sensitive to dietary requirements and could modify dishes to suit your requirements.

7. Make a Safe Snacking Plan: If you know you'll be hungry before your dinner comes or if dining out would require a longer wait, think about packing a little, IC-friendly snack to satisfy your hunger.

8. Be Educated about Trigger Foods: Learn about common meals that cause IC, such as citrus, tomatoes, and spicy foods. This information aids in your decision-making when perusing the menu.

9. Be Firm but Polite: When expressing your dietary requirements, it's important to be firm, but don't forget to be kind. The majority of restaurants make an effort to satisfy patron preferences, and efficient communication facilitates this process.

It may take a little more work for you to eat out when you have interstitial cystitis, but you may still enjoy restaurant meals without endangering the health of your bladder with planning and communication.

CHAPTER 9: MANAGING IC IN DIFFERENT LIFE STAGES

Interstitial cystitis, often known as IC, is a disorder that can afflict people at various phases of their lives, beginning with pregnancy and continuing through childhood and even into their senior years. To properly manage symptoms, it is essential to navigate the food choices that are available during these periods. Within the scope of this chapter, we will investigate nutrition techniques that are suitable for pregnant women who have interstitial cystitis (IC), cover nutrition for older citizens who are managing IC, and address issues for children who have IC.

IC-Friendly Pregnancy Nutrition

A unique and important stage of life is pregnancy, and controlling IC during this time necessitates paying close attention to diet. Although every pregnancy is unique, pregnant moms should take into account the following IC-friendly eating guidelines:

1. Hydration is Key: Maintaining enough hydration is critical for both pregnant women and those who have IC. Herbal teas, coconut water, and water infusions can all help you stay hydrated without making your IC symptoms worse.

2. Select Low-Acid Meals: To lessen the chance of inducing IC symptoms, choose low-acid foods. Eat a diet high in healthy grains,

lean meats, and veggies that are easy on the bladder.

3. Include Nutrients That Are Safe for Pregnancy:

Make sure you're getting the necessary nutrients, such as folic acid, iron, calcium, and omega-3 fatty acids, for a healthy pregnancy. Think about foods that are high in nutrients, such as fatty fish, leafy greens, lean meats, and dairy products.

4. Keep an Eye on Your Caffeine Intake: Although moderate caffeine use is typically seen as safe during pregnancy, it's important to keep an eye on how it affects your symptoms of IC. Reducing caffeine intake may be beneficial if it aggravates symptoms.

5. Recognize and Steer Clear of Trigger Foods: Certain foods have the potential to exacerbate symptoms of IC. Citrus fruits, tomatoes, and spicy meals are common triggers. Keeping a meal journal could assist in identifying particular triggers.

6. Create Well-Balanced Meals: Create meals that are well-balanced and incorporate a range of foods and macronutrients. By doing this, you can minimize the chance of symptom flare-ups while still ensuring that your nutritional needs are met.

7. Communicate with Healthcare Professionals: Keep your healthcare practitioner informed about your dietary requirements and any difficulties you may be

having regularly. They can offer advice suited to your particular circumstance.

Pregnancy-related IC management entails striking a balance between the mother's and the child's dietary demands and being aware of possible triggers.

Children and Interstitial Cystitis

Any age can be affected by interstitial cystitis, especially young children. Even though IC is less frequent in younger populations, parents, medical professionals, and the child must work together to manage the kid's symptoms. The following things to think about if your kid has interstitial cystitis:

1. Communication is Key: When dealing with older children who can voice their symptoms and preferences, it is extremely important to have open and honest communication. Urge your youngster to report any discomfort or symptom changes.

2. Recognize Trigger Items: Assist your kid in identifying foods that might exacerbate symptoms. Maintain a diet journal and record

any associations you find between particular foods and relapses of symptoms.

3. Establish a Helpful Environment: Promote a helpful atmosphere both at home and at school. Inform caregivers and educators about your child's nutritional needs so they can offer suitable alternatives.

4. Select IC-Friendly Snacks: For school meals and after-school pleasures, select IC-friendly snacks. Add less likely-to-cause-symptom foods like yogurt, fresh produce, whole-grain snacks, and fruits.

5. Promote Hydration: Watch out for your child's fluid intake, since this is essential for controlling IC symptoms. Include water or IC-friendly drinks in their regular regimen.

6. Provide Balanced Meals: Make meals that are balanced by including a range of foods from various dietary categories. Incorporate lean meats, healthy grains, and bladder-friendly veggies into their diet.

7. Work with Healthcare Providers: To develop a thorough management strategy, and cooperate with healthcare providers. They can provide advice on food plans, prescription drugs, and other treatments that might help control symptoms.

Children with IC require a comprehensive management strategy that takes into account both environmental and nutritional aspects. Collaboration and open communication with healthcare providers are essential elements of efficient management.

Nutrition for Seniors with IC

There can be particular difficulties in treating interstitial cystitis as people age. Dietary decisions are vital to sustaining general health, and seniors may have extra health concerns. The following dietary tips are for elders who are controlling IC:

1. Attend to Particular Nutritional Demands: Seniors may have particular nutritional needs, such as higher calcium and vitamin D levels for healthy bones. Make the IC-friendly diet fit these particular needs.

2. Adapt to Changing Appetites: As people become older, their appetites could alter. Be flexible when it comes to taste preferences and provide a range of IC-friendly solutions to suit a variety of tastes.

3. Handle Medication Interactions: Elderly people may take several medications, some of which may interfere with particular meals. Consult your doctor frequently about prescription lists to make sure they're in line with an IC-friendly diet.

4. Pay Attention to Hydration: Elderly people may be more susceptible to dehydration, which can worsen symptoms of IC. Promote drinking water regularly and incorporate foods that are high in water content, including fruits and vegetables.

5. Take into Account Texture Modifications: Take into account changing the texture of foods for elderly people who might have trouble chewing or swallowing. Select gentler

options, but make sure they complement IC-friendly selections.

6. Keep an eye out for dietary sensitivities: As we age, our bodies may respond differently to certain foods. To reduce symptom flare-ups, keep an eye out for any new food sensitivities and modify the diet accordingly.

7. Give Nutrient-Dense Meals Priority: Give nutrient-dense foods priority to satisfy nutritional requirements while maintaining reasonable quantities. Lean meats, nutritious grains, and an assortment of vibrant fruits and vegetables may all be included in this.

8. Maintain Contact with Healthcare Professionals: To address any changes in symptoms or health status, schedule regular consultations with healthcare professionals. They can guarantee that nutritional requirements are satisfied and offer advice on dietary adjustments.

Taking into account the unique requirements and difficulties of aging is essential to managing IC in elders. Seniors may maintain bladder health and general well-being by being proactive and modifying the IC-friendly diet to suit specific health factors.

CHAPTER 10: BEYOND THE KITCHEN - LIFESTYLE TIPS

Managing interstitial cystitis (IC) involves more than just making changes to one's diet. The management of stress, physical activity, and sleep are all lifestyle factors that have a significant impact on determining the symptoms and general well-being of an individual. The purpose of this chapter is to provide folks with lifestyle advice that goes beyond the kitchen to assist them in efficiently navigating and managing IC.

Stress Management and IC

It is well known that stress frequently sets off the symptoms of IC. The connection between stress and flare-ups emphasizes how crucial it is to apply stress-reduction strategies regularly. The following are some methods to lessen stress and lessen its effects on IC:

1. Mindfulness Meditation: This technique for lowering stress and encouraging relaxation is concentrating on the here and now. Regularly practicing mindfulness can help reduce stress and anxiety.

2. Deep Breathing Activities: The body's relaxation response may be triggered by deep breathing exercises like diaphragmatic breathing. When under stress, use deep breathing exercises to help you feel calmer.

3. Progressive Muscle Relaxation (PMR): PMR includes gradually tensing and then relaxing different muscle groups to alleviate physical stress. Frequent practice can help reduce stress in general.

4. Yoga for Relaxation: Including a light yoga practice in your regimen will help your body and mind. Breathwork in conjunction with yoga positions can help promote relaxation and stress reduction.

5. Expressive Writing: Keeping a journal in which one records ideas and feelings can be a therapeutic method of managing stress. Expressive writing enables people to examine and let go of emotions, which may lessen the effect of those emotions on IC symptoms.

6. Make Self-Care a Priority: Take part in enjoyable and calming activities. Setting aside time for self-care, whether it be reading, taking a bath, or going outside, is crucial for stress management.

7. Seek Support: Make connections with a network of people who can help you, such as friends, family, or IC support groups. Getting assistance and exchanging experiences might help you manage your stress.

Through the integration of stress management strategies into their everyday lives, people with intermittent cystic fever (IC) can foster a more encouraging atmosphere that may help alleviate symptoms.

Exercise and Interstitial Cystitis

Regular physical activity is a cornerstone of general health, but persons with IC may question how exercise affects their symptoms. The following are things to think about and pointers for integrating exercise into an IC-friendly lifestyle:

1. Low-Impact Exercise Options: Choose exercises that are easy on the pelvic floor and bladder. In general, activities like swimming, walking, and stationary cycling are well tolerated.

2. Pelvic Floor Exercises: People with IC may benefit from strengthening their pelvic floor muscles. Exercises for the pelvic floor, commonly referred to as Kegel exercises, can enhance bladder health and muscular tone.

3. Gradual Progression: If you've been inactive, begin your workout regimen gradually. To prevent aggravating symptoms, start with brief workouts and progressively increase in time and intensity.

4. Stay Hydrated: It's important to stay properly hydrated when exercising, but people with IC need to be careful about how much fluid they consume. Sip water throughout the day and try hydrating with IC-friendly beverages.

5. Select Supportive Apparel: To reduce discomfort during exercise, wear loose-fitting, comfortable clothes and supportive undergarments. Fabrics that wick away moisture can assist in controlling perspiration and avoid discomfort.

6. Listen to Your Body: Observe how exercise affects your body. If some activities make your symptoms worse, change your routine or look into more tolerable options for exercise.

7. Include Relaxation Techniques: You could want to include deep breathing exercises or mindfulness exercises in your regimen after working out. This can assist in offsetting any symptom-related effects of stress.

8. Speak with Healthcare Professionals: See your healthcare providers before beginning a new fitness regimen. In addition to offering advice on activities that are appropriate for your particular circumstances, they could, if necessary, recommend you to a physical therapist.

Frequent exercise can improve general well-being and perhaps lessen the symptoms of IC when done carefully and according to each person's needs.

Sleep and IC Symptoms

A good night's sleep is essential for good health, and irregular sleep patterns can exacerbate the symptoms of IC. Here are some suggestions to help people with interstitial cystitis sleep better:

1. Create a Regular Sleep Schedule: Even on weekends, go to bed and wake up at the same time every day. Maintaining consistency can enhance the quality of sleep and support the body's internal clock.

2. Establish a Calm Bedtime Habit: Establish a peaceful nighttime routine to let your body know when it's time to unwind. This might be reading, doing light stretching, or using relaxation techniques.

3. Optimize Sleep Environment: Maintain a cool, calm, and dark bedroom to create a good sleeping environment. To improve comfort, spend money on pillows and a sturdy mattress.

4. Restrict Stimulants Before Bed: Refrain from using stimulants like caffeine and nicotine in the hours before bed. Certain drugs may make it difficult to fall asleep.

5. Control Fluid Consumption Before Bed: Although being hydrated is important, you should think about controlling your fluid consumption in the evening to reduce the need for late-night toilet breaks. Be aware of beverages that are IC-friendly.

6. Manage Stress and Anxiety: Use stress-reduction strategies to deal with any worry or tension that could interfere with your ability to sleep. This might entail mindfulness activities, meditation, or deep breathing.

7. Minimize Screen Time Before Bed: Limit your time spent in front of computers or phones before night. The body's regular sleep-wake cycle may be disrupted by the blue light that screens emit.

8. Speak with Healthcare Professionals: If sleep issues continue, speak with healthcare professionals to determine any possible underlying reasons. They might provide direction on tactics or remedies to raise the quality of sleep.

Setting aside time for a restful night's sleep is crucial for controlling IC symptoms and enhancing general health and well-being.

APPENDIX

In the process of controlling Interstitial Cystitis (IC), useful materials and tools can be very helpful. A meal diary template is included in this appendix to assist in leading a conscious and bladder-friendly lifestyle.

Food Diary Template

For people with IC, keeping a food diary is an effective way to monitor their nutritional intake, symptoms, and possible triggers. Making thorough notes on everything you eat and drink, as well as any related symptoms, can help you see trends and make well-informed dietary decisions. A thorough food diary template to help you with this procedure is provided below:

Date: __________

Meal or Snack: ______________________________

Beverages: ________________________________

Symptoms   (if   any):

____

____

Food and Beverage Details:

Breakfast:

Item 1: ______________________________

Item 2: ______________________________

Item 3: ______________________________

Mid-Morning Snack:

Item 1: ______________________________

Item 2: ______________________________

Item 3: ______________________________

Lunch:

Item 1: _______________________________________

Item 2: _______________________________________

Item 3: _______________________________________

Afternoon Snack:

Item 1: _______________________________________

Item 2: _______________________________________

Item 3: _______________________________________

Dinner:

Item 1: _______________________________________

Item 2: _______________________________________

Item 3: _______________________________________

Evening Snack:

Item 1: _______________________________________

Item 2: _______________________________________

Item 3: ______________________________________

Beverages:

Beverage 1: ___________________________________

Beverage 2: ___________________________________

Beverage 3: ___________________________________

Symptoms:

Bladder Discomfort/Pain (0-10 scale): _______

Frequency of Urination: _______ times

Intensity   of   Symptoms
(Mild/Moderate/Severe): _______

Any   Additional   Notes:

____

____

____

____

____

By regularly using this template, you can find patterns and correlations between particular meals and drinks and your symptoms of IC. Before analyzing trends and modifying your diet, it's best to keep the journal filled out for a minimum of one to two weeks.